# PROLACTINOMAS and PREGNANCY

# PROLACTINOMAS
# and PREGNANCY

The Proceedings of a Special Symposium held at the XIth World Congress
on Fertility and Sterility, Dublin, June 1983

Symposium Editor: H. S. Jacobs

General Congress Editors:
R. F. Harrison,
J. Bonnar and W. Thompson

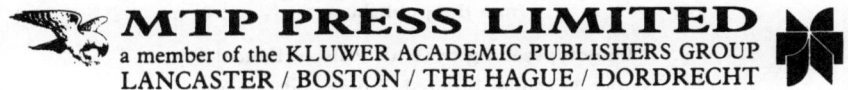
MTP PRESS LIMITED
a member of the KLUWER ACADEMIC PUBLISHERS GROUP
LANCASTER / BOSTON / THE HAGUE / DORDRECHT

Published in the UK and Europe by
MTP Press Limited
Falcon House
Lancaster, England

**British Library Cataloguing in Publication Data**

Prolactinomas and pregnancy.
1. Prolactinoma—Congresses
I. Jacobs, H. S. II. World Congress on Fertility and Sterility (*11th: 1983: Dublin*)
616.99'247  RC280.P5

Published in the USA by
MTP Press
A division of Kluwer Boston Inc
190 Old Derby Street
Hingham, MA 02043, USA

**Library of Congress Cataloging in Publication Data**

Main entry under title:
Prolactinomas and Pregnancy.
  Bibliography: P.
  Includes index.
  1. Infertility, female – Congresses. 2. Pregnancy, complications of – Congresses. 3. Prolactinoma – Congresses. I. Jacobs, H. S. (Howard Saul). II. Harrison, R. F. (Robert Frederick). III. Bonnar, John. IV. Thompson, W. M. World congress on fertility and sterility (11th: 1983: Dublin, Dublin)
  [DNLM: 1. Prolactin – secretion – Congresses. 2. Pituitary neoplasms – secretion – Congresses. 3. Pituitary neoplasms – in pregnancy – Congresses. 4. Infertility, female – etiology – Congresses. 5. Infertility, female – therapy – Congresses. WK 515 P9646 1983]
  RG201.P76 1983          618.1'78          83-22259

  ISBN-13: 978-94-011-6357-6    e-ISBN-13: 978-94-011-6355-2
  DOI: 10.1007/978-94-011-6355-2

Phototypesetting by Titus Wilson, Kendal

Butler & Tanner Limited, Frome and London

# Contents

List of Contributors                                                    7

1   Introduction: prolactinomas and pregnancy
    H. S. Jacobs                                                        9

2   Medical investigation of abnormal prolactin states
    P. G. Crosignani, C. Ferrari, P. Rampini, P. Adelasco,
    C. Zavaglia, G. Brambilla, M. Boghen and A. Paracchi              13

3   Neuroradiology of prolactinomas
    K. Hall                                                           21

4   The outcome of pituitary exploration in patients with
    hyperprolactinaemic infertility
    G. Teasdale, A. Richards, R. Bullock and J. Thomson               33

5   Medical treatment of prolactinomas
    S. Franks and H. S. Jacobs                                        39

6   Surveillance of Parlodel (bromocriptine) in pregnancy and
    offspring
    P. Krupp and I. Turkalj                                           45

7   Prolactinomas in pregnancy
    T. Bergh and S. J. Nillius                                        51

Index                                                                 57

# List of Contributors

**P. ADELASCO**
III Department of Obstetrics and
  Gynecology
University of Milan
Via M. Melloni, 52
20120 Milano
Italy

**T. BERGH**
Department of Obstetrics and
  Gynecology
University Hospital
S-751 85 Uppsala
Sweden

**M. BOGHEN**
II Department of Medicine
Fatebenefratelli Hospital
Corso di Porta Nuova, 23
20121 Milano
Italy

**G. BRAMBILLA**
III Department of Obstetrics and
  Gynecology
University of Milan
Via M. Melloni, 52
20129 Milano
Italy

**R. BULLOCK**
Institute of Neurological Sciences
Southern General Hospital
Glasgow G51 4TF
UK

**P. CROSIGNANI**
III Department of Obstetrics and
  Gynecology
University of Milan
Via M. Melloni, 52
20129 Milano
Italy

**C. FERRARI**
II Department of Medicine
Fatebenefratelli Hospital
Corso di Porta Nuova, 23
20121 Milano
Italy

**S. FRANKS**
Department of Obstetrics and
  Gynaecology
St. Marys Hospital Medical School
London W2 1PG
UK

**K. HALL**
Department of Neuroradiology
Regional Neurological Centre
Newcastle General Hospital
Westgate Road
Newcastle upon Tyne
Tyne and Wear NE4 6BE
UK

**H. S. JACOBS**
Department of Endocrinology
Middlesex Hospital
Mortimer Street
London W1P 7PN
UK

PROLACTINOMAS AND PREGNANCY

P. KRUPP
Pharmaceutical Department
Clinical Research
Drug Monitoring Centre
Sandoz Ltd.
CH-4002 Basle
Switzerland

S. J. NILLIUS
Department of Obstetrics and
  Gynaecology
University Hospital
S-751 85 Uppsala
Sweden

A. PARACCHI
II Department of Medicine
Fatebenefratelli Hospital
Corso di Porta Nuova, 23
20121 Milano
Italy

P. RAMPINI
II Department of Medicine
Fatebenefratelli Hospital
Corso di Porta Nuova 23
20121 Milano
Italy

A. RICHARDS
Institute of Neurological Sciences
Southern General Hospital
Glasgow G51 4TF
UK

G. TEASDALE
Department of Neurosurgery
Institute of Neurological Sciences
Southern General Hospital
Glasgow G51 4TF
UK

J. THOMSON
Institute of Neurological Sciences
Southern General Hospital
Glasgow G51 4TF
UK

I. TURKALJ
Pharmaceutical Department
Clinical Research
Drug Monitoring Centre
Sandoz Ltd.
CH-4002 Basle
Switzerland

C. ZAVAGLIA
III Department of Obstetrics and
  Gynecology
University of Milan
Via M. Melloni 52
20129 Milano
Italy

# 1
# Introduction: prolactinomas and pregnancy

H. S. JACOBS

---

The last decade has seen a revolution in the treatment of anovulatory infertility and nowhere has this been more obvious than in the diagnosis and management of patients with hyperprolactinaemia. Notwithstanding the remarkable increase in our understanding of the neuropharmacological control of prolactin secretion (detailed by Dr Crosignani in the opening chapter of this book), the single most reliable diagnostic guide to a disturbance of prolactin secretion remains the basal serum prolactin concentration. While much confusion and uncertainty exists in the exact interpretation of the normal range, the simple point to remember is that with prolactin concentrations, as with all clinical investigations, correct evaluation demands that one takes into account the clinical context in which the measurement is made. Thus because it is known that oestrogen stimulates prolactin release and that women with amenorrhoea due to hyperprolactinaemia suffer from oestrogen deficiency, a minor elevation of the serum prolactin concentration in an oestrogen deficient patient with amenorrhoea is of much greater clinical significance than a considerable elevation in a well oestrogenized patient with an intact menstrual cycle.

At least half the women presenting with hyperprolactinaemic amenorrhoea have a prolactin-secreting pituitary tumour (prolactinoma). The exact proportion diagnosed depends upon the imaging procedure used and Dr Hall outlines with great clarity the information that can be obtained from the various procedures presently in use (Chapter 3). The advantages of CT scanning, in which the pituitary itself rather than its bony carapace is imaged, are clearly described. In addition Dr Hall describes the advantages of the direct coronal scan compared with multiple axial scans with computer reconstructions in the coronal and sagittal planes. This is a fascinating article in which the limits of current radiological techniques are also drawn.

Several modalities of treatment exist, but undoubtedly surgical extirpation and medical treatment with bromocriptine are the two most frequently used. Professor Teasdale and colleagues (Chapter 4) address the type of clinical information endocrinologists and gynaecologists find particularly helpful. Thus in contrast to the majority of articles by surgeons, this chapter describes the outcome both in terms of rates of normalization of prolactin concentrations and in terms of pregnancy rates. He shows that in experienced hands surgical removal of prolactinomas confined to the pituitary fossa continues to provide a reliable method of treatment, with a remarkably low rate of endocrine (and indeed surgical) complications.

Drs Franks and Jacobs describe some aspects of the use of dopaminergic agonists (Chapter 5). In addition to describing the familiar story of the success of bromocriptine in normalizing prolactin secretion and reconstituting fertility, they provide long-term follow-up data on patients originally treated with bromocriptine 6–8 years ago. Naturally such data are only now becoming available and for some patients the picture is looking quite optimistic, even for long-term remission of symptoms in patients who have discontinued their medical therapy.

Drs Bergh and Nillius deal directly with the problem of the prolactinoma that expands during pregnancy (Chapter 7). In fact, it turns out that this is a rare problem. At first it seems remarkable that a complication we all worried about so much should not eventuate, or only so as a rarity. In my opinion the reason is the remarkable shrinkage of prolactin-secreting pituitary tumours that occurs on treatment with bromocriptine. As described by Franks and Jacobs, the tumour quite rapidly shrinks away from the walls of the expanded fossa and so any tendency for it to enlarge during pregnancy can be readily accommodated. Of course, in the past, when ovulation was induced with drugs that were not dopaminergic agonists, such shrinkage did not occur and therefore room had not been made for pituitary

10

expansion during pregnancy, a phenomenon that of course occurs normally. Should clinical symptoms of pituitary expansion occur in a patient with a prolactinoma (whether or not she was originally treated with bromocriptine) it does seem, however, that using bromocriptine during pregnancy is safe to both mother and fetus, based upon the excellent report of the extensive post-marketing surveillance of the use of bromocriptine in pregnancy reported by Drs Krupp and Turkalj (page 45).

In conclusion the following chapters describe most aspects of the management of patients with prolactinomas in relation to their infertility and their progress through pregnancy. I commend them to you as up-to-date accounts by experienced authors of problems faced by all clinicians treating this common condition.

# 2
# Medical investigation of abnormal prolactin states

P. G. CROSIGNANI, C. FERRARI, P. RAMPINI,
P. ADELASCO, C. ZAVAGLIA, G. BRAMBILLA,
M. BOGHEN and A. PARACCHI

In hyperprolactinaemic patients, despite the large amount of clinical data, radiological studies and biochemical testing, the most useful diagnostic criteria remain the basal serum prolactin (PRL) levels and the results of radiological investigation of the sella and suprasellar region. High-resolution CT scans are especially helpful. These statements are supported by our experience with several diagnostic tests of prolactin secretion, which have been carried out in a large population of hyperprolactinaemic subjects over the last 7 years.

## PATIENTS AND METHODS

Patients with hyperprolactinaemia of different origin have been studied for basal serum PRL determination, radiological studies of the sella and in most cases for different functional tests of PRL secretion. On the basis of clinical and radiological findings, patients' conditions have been classified as follows:

(1) Idiopathic hyperprolactinaemia, when conventional tomography and CT scans of the sella and suprasellar region were normal.

(2) Microprolactinoma, by the presence of typical radiological

13

findings; surgical confirmation has been subsequently obtained in the 30 patients undergoing operation.

(3) Macroprolactinoma, on the basis of CT-scan findings.
(4) Acromegaly, as shown by concomitant GH and PRL hypersecretion; all these patients had evidence of pituitary macroadenoma.
(5) Empty sella syndrome, as diagnosed by CT scans.
(6) Hypothalamic lesions, as suggested by CT scan and confirmed by surgery.
(7) Uraemia; these patients were studied during chronic haemodialysis.

The following functional tests were used:

(1) TRH test ($200 \mu$g i.v.). Individual responses were classified as normal when the maximum increase over baseline was in the range of normal subjects, as absent when this increase was less than 50%, and as impaired when the increase was greater than 50% but below the normal range.
(2) Sulpiride (100 mg i.m.) or domperidone (2 or 8 mg i.v.) test. The criteria for judging the individual responses were also derived from parallel studies in control subjects, with definition of normal, absent or impaired responses as for the TRH test.
(3) Directly acting dopamine agonists or dopamine precursors:
    (a) dopamine ($5 \mu$g kg$^{-1}$ min$^{-1}$ infused i.v. during 120 min),
    (b) L-dopa (500 mg by mouth),
    (c) bromocriptine (2.5 mg by mouth),
    (d) dihydroergocristine (6 mg by mouth).
    The criterion for a normal response was a lowering of PRL value to below 50% of the baseline concentration after either dopamine, L-dopa or bromocriptine. Dihydroergocristine was observed not to lower PRL levels significantly in normal subjects at this dose when given by mouth[1].
(4) Central nervous system acting dopaminergic drugs:
    (a) L-dopa (100 mg by mouth) plus carbidopa (35 mg by mouth) after pretreatment with carbidopa 50 mg by mouth six hourly for four doses,
    (b) nomifensine (200 mg by mouth).
    The criteria for a normal response were PRL lowering to below

14

50% of baseline after carbidopa plus L-dopa, or to below 65% of baseline after nomifensine.

## RESULTS AND DISCUSSION

Basal PRL levels in the various categories of hyperprolactinaemic patients examined are reported in Figure 1, showing that values

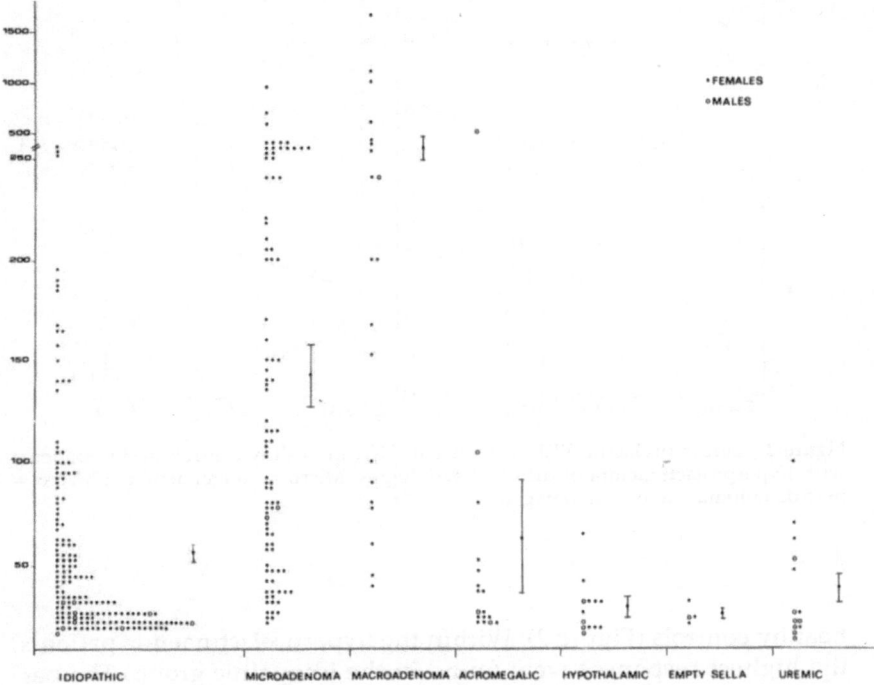

**Figure 1**  Basal serum prolactin concentrations in individual subjects with hyperprolactinaemia of different aetiology. Mean ±SE values are also shown

above 200 ng ml$^{-1}$ are almost solely found in patients with prolactinoma. This is in agreement with many previous studies, but much overlap exists between the different aetiologies.

## TRH test

The mean PRL response observed in the various groups of patients was always significantly lower, on a percent basis, than that of

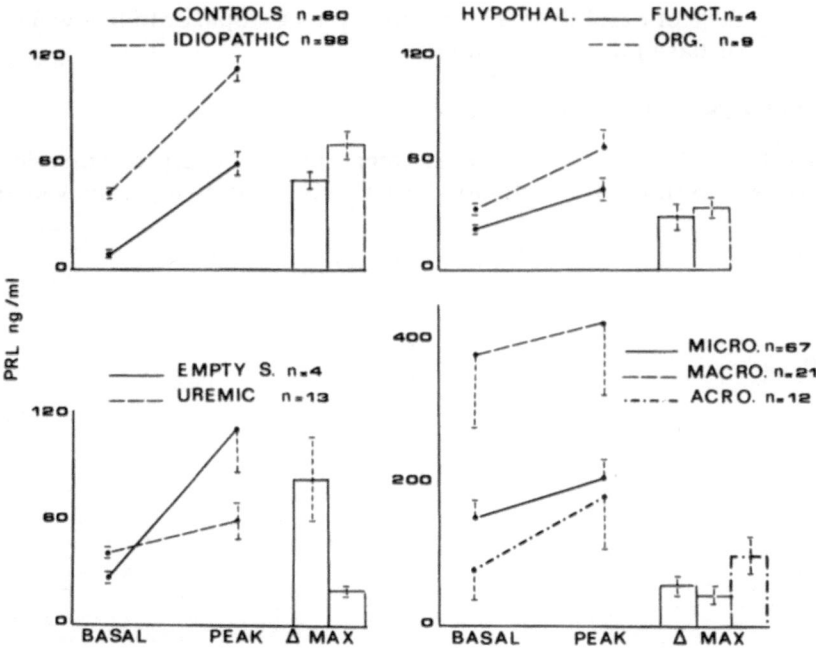

**Figure 2** Serum prolactin (PRL) response to TRH in healthy controls and in patients with hyperprolactinaemia of different aetiologies. Micro = microadenoma; Macro = macroadenoma; Acro = acromegaly

healthy controls (Figure 2). Within the hyperprolactinaemic patients, the highest responses were found in the idiopathic group. The patterns of PRL response to TRH in 228 hyperprolactinaemic subjects indicate that most but not all patients with prolactinoma or with uraemia do not adequately respond to the stimulus; a large overlap between groups is, however, evident.

## Sulpiride and domperidone tests

Both these antidopaminergic drugs elicited normal PRL responses in many patients with idiopathic hyperprolactinaemia but only in a few with prolactinoma. It is noteworthy that none of the 19 subjects with hypothalamic disease or acromegaly responded adequately to dopamine receptor blockade[2]. An important finding was the normal PRL response obtained in five patients with radiological evidence of microprolactinoma, in two of whom the diagnosis was confirmed at surgery.

Since exogenous dopamine infusion restores the normal PRL response to sulpiride in unresponsive subjects with either idiopathic, adenomatous or hypothalamic hyperprolactinaemia[3] a defective concentration of dopamine at the lactotrophs seems to be the cause of the failure of dopamine antagonists to stimulate PRL secretion in these patients.

Some interesting information may be derived by comparing the responses to TRH and sulpiride tests in the same hyperprolactinaemic subjects. In fact a higher PRL increase is elicited by sulpiride than TRH in patients with idiopathic hyperprolactinaemia as well as in the controls, while prolactinoma patients appear unresponsive to both stimuli, and those with hypothalamic disease show a positive response to TRH associated with an absent response to sulpiride. These data suggest that the combination of the two tests may be of some practical value in subjects with mild to moderate hyperprolactinaemia and no radiological evidence of pituitary adenoma[4].

## Direct dopamine agonists or precursors

All of the three substances used (dopamine, L-dopa and bromocriptine) induced a substantial lowering of PRL value in most patients irrespective of the underlying aetiology, as previously reported[5]. However, a certain proportion of subjects showed partial or total resistance to the drugs; this is reminiscent of the findings obtained with chronic bromocriptine treatment[5].

This resistance to dopamine action may be caused either by defective dopamine receptors at the lactotrophs or by a postreceptor defect[6]. Nevertheless, compared with the relatively uncommon dopamine resistance, the large majority of hyperprolactinaemic patients are responsive, or even hyper-responsive, to the action of dopamine. This is suggested by the recent finding that an oral dose of the relatively weak dopamine agonist dihydroergocristine can suppress PRL levels significantly in hyperprolactinaemic states of different aetiology but not in healthy controls[1]. These data are reminiscent of previous findings obtained with subemetic doses of apomorphine[7].

17

## Central nervous system acting dopaminergic drugs

Most patients in the various groups had an impaired or absent suppression of PRL in both the carbidopa plus L-dopa and the nomifensine tests, as previously reported[8].

The failure of nomifensine administration to lower PRL levels in most hyperprolactinaemic patients was initially attributed to defective activation of brain dopaminergic pathways in these subjects[8,9]. However, the recent finding that nomifensine elevates serum growth hormone (GH) levels in hyperprolactinaemic as well as in healthy subjects[10,11] makes this hypothesis unlikely and suggests that the impairment lies in the dopamine transport to the lactotrophs, prob-

**Table 1** Prevalence (expressed as percentages) of: (A) Pituitary dopamine resistance*, (B) Pituitary dopamine concentration defect[†], and (C) CNS dopamine inhibition defect[‡]. Number of subjects tested is given in parenthesies

| Group | Idiopathic hyperpro- lactinaemia | Micro- prolactinoma | Macro- prolactinoma | Acromegaly | Hypo- thalamic hyperpro- lactinaemia |
|-------|----------------------------------|---------------------|---------------------|------------|--------------------------------------|
| A | 17 (54) | 15 (59) | 33 (18) | 0 (7) | 0 (7) |
| B | 38 (50) | 92 (58) | 100 (19) | 100 (8) | 100 (11) |
| C | 70 (34) | 82 (24) | 80 (20) | 50 (4) | 75 (4) |

*As assessed by impaired PRL inhibition by dopamine, L-dopa or bromocriptine.
[†]As assessed by impaired PRL stimulation by sulpiride or domperidone.
[‡]As assessed by impaired PRL inhibition by carbidopa plus L-dopa or nomifensine.

ably due to alterations in the microcirculation. Table 1 summarizes the prevalence of the three dopaminergic defects discussed above in the different groups of hyperprolactinaemic patients we have studied. These data show that dopamine resistance is relatively uncommon in hyperprolactinaemia, while evidence of pituitary dopamine deficiency is quite common and almost uniformly found in patients with prolactinoma. These conclusions are in contrast with reports suggesting that dopaminergic tone is increased in hyperprolactinaemia on the basis of thyrotrophin (TSH) hyper-responsiveness to dopamine antagonists[12] and that hyperprolactinaemic subjects may be more resistant to the PRL-lowering effect of dopamine infusion than healthy controls[13]. The results of TSH testing, however, cannot simply be extrapolated to the PRL secretion system, and different results have been obtained with dopamine infusion by other groups with both *in vivo* and *in vitro* experiments[6,14]. These discrepancies probably result from the small number of patients studied and from the variable prevalence of subjects truly resistant to the action of dopamine in the different investigations. This is a particularly important bias in studies like that of Bansal *et al.*[13], which were performed in a small number of subjects.

## Acknowledgements

This work was supported in part by C.N.R. Special Program 'Control of Neoplastic Growth'.

## References

1. Ferrari, C., Romussi, M., Benco, R., Rampini, P. and Mailland, F. (1983). Effect of dihydroergocristine administration on serum prolactin and growth hormone levels in normal, hyperprolactinemic, and acromegalic subjects: further evidence for pituitary dopamine deficiency in these conditions. *Acta Endocrinol.*, **103**, 1
2. Ferrari, C., Scarduelli, C., Rampini, P. *et al.* (1983). Prolactin response to the dopamine antagonists sulpiride and domperidone: further evidence for pituitary dopamine deficiency in hyperprolactinemic disorders of different etiology. *Gynecol. Obstet. Invest.* (In press)
3. Crosignani, P. G., Reschini, E., Peracchi, M., Lombroso, G. C., Mattei, A. and Caccamo, A. (1977). Failure of dopamine infusion to suppress the plasma prolactin response to sulpiride in normal and hyperprolactinemic subjects. *J. Clin. Endocrinol. Metab.*, **45**, 841
4. Ferrari, C., Rampini, P., Benco, R., Caldara, R., Scarduelli, C. and Crosignani, P. G. (1982). Functional characterization of hypothalamic hyperprolactinemia. *J. Clin. Endocrinol. Metab.*, **55**, 897
5. Crosignani, P. G., Ferrari, C., Liuzzi, A., *et al.* (1982). Treatment of hyperprolactinemic states with different drugs: a study with bromocriptine, metergoline, and lisuride. *Fertil. Steril.*, **37**, 61
6. Bethea, C. L., Ramsdell, J. S., Jaffe, R. B., Wilson, C. B. and Weiner, R. I. (1982). Characterization of the dopaminergic regulation of human prolactin-secreting cells cultured on extracellular matrix. *J. Clin. Endocrinol. Metab.*, **54**, 893
7. Martin, J. B., Lal, S., Tolis, G. and Friesen, H. G. (1974). Inhibition by apomorphine of prolactin secretion in patients with elevated serum prolactin. *J. Clin. Endocrinol. Metab.*, **39**, 180
8. Crosignani, P. G., Ferrari, C., Malinverni, A., Barbieri, C., Mattei, A., Caldara, R. and Rocchetti, M. (1980). Effect of central nervous system dopaminergic activation on prolactin secretion in man: evidence for a common central defect in hyperprolactinemic patients with and without radiological signs of pituitary tumors. *J. Clin. Endocrinol. Metab.*, **51**, 1068
9. Müller, E. E., Genazzani, A. R. and Murru, S. (1978). Nomifensine diagnostic test in hyperprolactinemic states. *J. Clin. Endocrinol. Metab.*, **47**, 1352
10. Dallabonzana, D., Spelta, B., Botalla, L. *et al.* (1982). Effects of nomifensine on growth hormone and prolactin secretion in normal subjects and in pathological hyperprolactinemia. *J. Clin. Endocrinol. Metab.*, **54**, 1125
11. Ferrari, C., Caldara, R., Barbieri, C. *et al.* (1981). Central nervous system and

pituitary mechanisms in dopaminergic stimulation of growth hormone release in women. *Neuroendocrinology*, **32**, 213

12. Scanlon, M. F., Rodriguez-Arnao, M. D., McGregor, A. M. *et al.* (1981). Altered dopaminergic regulation of thyrotrophin release in patients with prolactinomas: comparison with other tests of hypothalamic-pituitary function. *Clin. Endocrinol.*, **14**, 133
13. Bansal, S., Lee, L. A. and Woolf, P. D. (1981). Abnormal prolactin responsivity to dopaminergic suppression in hyperprolactinemic patients. *Am. J. Med.*, **71**, 961
14. Reschini, E., Ferrari, C., Peracchi, M., Fadini, R., Meschia, M. and Crosignani, P. G. (1980). Effect of dopamine infusion on serum prolactin concentration in normal and hyperprolactinemic subjects. *Clin. Endocrinol.*, **13**, 519

# 3
# Neuroradiology of prolactinomas

K. HALL

The neuroradiological methods that can be used in the detection and delineation of known or suspected prolactinomas are numerous. They include relatively non-invasive techniques such as skull radiography, sellar tomography and CT scanning. Sometimes more invasive procedures are deemed to be necessary, such as cerebral angiography, basal cisternography and cavernous sinus venography.

## FACTORS INFLUENCING THE CHOICE OF NEURORADIOLOGICAL TECHNIQUES

The decision as to which of these methods should be used in any individual case will depend on several factors. The first is the skill and expertise of the radiologists, allied to the sophistication of the apparatus that they have available. One important point is that all of the invasive methods mentioned above are potentially dangerous and may, in some circumstances, be avoided if a third- or fourth-generation CT scanner is in use.

The second factor influencing the choice of radiological investigations is what sort of treatment will be used. Thus if medical treatment alone is to be used very little radiological investigation will be necessary. In our experience, all that is required prior to the initiation of bromocriptine therapy for prolactinomas is a plain radiograph of the skull to exclude a large tumour. If, however, the surgical removal of a prolactinoma is contemplated, either as the primary form of therapy or because bromocriptine has failed or has not been tolerated by the patient, then the surgeon may demand more information from the radiologist. He will probably wish to confirm the presence of a tumour in the gland and may want to know where it lies. In addition, if it is large he may wish to have some advance information about the precise relationships of the lesion to adjacent structures such as the optic nerves and chiasm and the carotid arteries and their branches. Some surgeons may wish to know about the anatomy of the cavernous sinuses, and their interconnections, prior to surgical exploration via the transsphenoidal route. The demand for such information will, obviously, depend on past experience during surgical exploration of the pituitary fossa.

The neuroradiological techniques that are thought necessary will also depend on the size of the prolactinoma. Pituitary adenomas are fairly arbitrarily divided into either microadenomas (diameter ⩽ 10 mm) or macroadenomas (diameter > 10 mm), the importance of this distinction being that microadenomas probably tend to become macroadenomas and that the smaller tumours are easier to remove, with less risk of recurrence. The one basic radiological difference between these two subdivisions of pituitary adenomas, and this applies to prolactinomas in particular, is that macroadenomas tend to enlarge the sella whereas the microadenomas do not. The large tumours tend to exert effects on adjacent structures, such as arteries and nerves, and to demonstrate these changes the invasive techniques may be necessary.

## THE DETECTION AND DELINEATION OF MACROPROLACTINOMAS

### Sellar radiography

As already mentioned, macroprolactinomas tend to enlarge the pituitary fossa and this can be readily assessed if it is fairly gross. However, if there is any doubt about sellar expansion an arbitrary method can be used to calculate the 'sellar volume'[1]. In this the length and height of the pituitary fossa are measured on the lateral film, and its width is determined from the posteroanterior (PA) film. These figures are multiplied together and then divided by two to arrive at this so-called volume, a figure of 1500 mm³ usually being taken as the upper limit of normal.

A pituitary adenoma is not the only cause of an enlarged sella. It can be enlarged by pressure from a dilated third ventricle in chronic hydrocephalus, by a craniopharyngioma or by a large intrasellar aneurysm. However, the commonest cause of an expanded sella turcica, after a pituitary adenoma, is an empty sella. This is the term used for an intrasellar arachnoid herniation in which a CSF-filled sac bulges downwards through a defect in the diaphragma sellae, into the fossa, causing compression of the pituitary gland as well as symmetrical, globular sellar enlargement.

A macroadenoma in the pituitary fossa is often not central in position and any enlargement will produce asymmetry and depression of the sellar floor. The floor will often become thinned and eroded and the tumour may bulge down into the sphenoidal sinus.

If a large adenoma grows upwards out of the pituitary fossa it will tend to distort the anterior clinoid processes and push the dorsum sellae backwards. Thus an erect dorsum sellae may indicate a fairly large suprasellar extension of the tumour. When the tumour becomes extremely large the dorsum sellae and the top of the clivus can be destroyed completely.

When the sella is definitely abnormal sellar tomography is rarely indicated. We only perform tomography in such circumstances if the surgeon wishes to see the sellar floor and the anatomy of the sphenoidal sinuses, prior to transsphenoidal surgery, if these have not been shown by the CT scan.

## CT scanning

When CT scanning was first introduced it rapidly became established as the next radiological investigation to carry out, after the initial skull radiograph, in the detection and delineation of pituitary adenomas. The older generations of scanners, by means of scans in the axial and coronal planes, could demonstrate very adequately large intrasellar tumours and those with extensions into the sphenoidal sinus and the suprasellar regions.

With these scanners pituitary tumours of all types tend to be slightly denser than surrounding brain and show fairly homogeneous enhancement, i.e. following the administration of intravenous contrast medium they appear whiter on the scans. Some tumours, however, show a more cystic or necrotic appearance, having a central darker area surrounded by an enhancing white ring.

A CT scan can also demonstrate, and sometimes distinguish from a pituitary adenoma, other lesions in or near the sella, such as a craniopharyngioma, a meningioma or a large aneurysm. An empty sella can often be suggested by the low CSF density in the sella, though sometimes a cystic or necrotic tumour produces a similar appearance and can be misdiagnosed as an empty sella.

CT scanning is of value in the follow-up of pituitary adenomas, whether they have been treated or not. Thus, a decrease in tumour size can be readily appreciated on repeat scans when a patient with a large prolactinoma is treated with bromocriptine, or other medical treatment.

Only fairly large tumours, and quite marked changes in tumour size, can be detected with these older CT scanners. A small macroadenoma, or other small lesion in the sellar region, can be missed, making other radiological methods such as basal cisternography necessary. The newer third- and fourth-generation scanners can, however, demonstrate these lesions much more reliably, as described later in the section on the CT scanning of microprolactinomas.

### Cerebral angiography

Bilateral carotid angiography may be demanded by the surgeon before surgical removal of a macroprolactinoma, by the transsphenoidal or the intracranial approach. This angiogram should show the relationship of the tumour to the adjacent arteries, which may be quite markedly distorted and displaced by a large tumour. Sometimes the adjacent artery may be encased by a prolactinoma, making removal impossible.

When a transsphenoidal approach is to be used the surgeon may want to know that the carotid arteries in the cavernous sinuses are not too tortuous and are not bulging into the pituitary gland. Also, he may wish to be certain that there are no small aneurysms arising from these arteries and bulging into the gland. These precautions should prevent disastrous arterial haemorrhage during the operation because; if an arterial anomaly is found, a different approach can be chosen.

Rarely, the angiogram may show that rare cause of an enlarged sella, a huge intrasellar aneurysm, another potentially dangerous lesion for the pituitary surgeon.

24

## Basal cisternography, with CT

In the basal cisternogram, a positive contrast medium, such as metrizamide or iopamidol, is introduced into the basal subarachnoid cisterns, especially those adjacent to the sella. These cisterns and their contents, normal or abnormal, are then visualized by lateral radiography or tomography and also by axial and coronal plane CT scanning. This technique was developed to supplement conventional CT scanning on the older generation scanners in an attempt to demonstrate smaller tumours, etc.[2].

The cisternogram should show quite small macroprolactinomas with small suprasellar extensions. It will also demonstrate the relationship of small or medium-sized tumours to the optic nerves and chiasm, which the surgeon may find of value at operation. An empty sella, be it large or small, can be readily demonstrated by this technique and small changes in prolactinoma size are easily seen[3]. If more sophisticated CT scanners are available basal cisternography is of more limited value.

## Cavernous sinus venography

In some centres cavernous sinus venography is used instead of carotid angiography to demonstrate arterial anomalies in the sellar region[4]. The carotid arteries show as filling defects in the opacified cavernous sinuses and anomalies such as tortuosity and aneurysms can be detected. Sometimes, however, an angiogram may still be required to confirm the abnormality shown on the venogram. The advantage of the venogram over the angiogram is that it is less invasive, it is simpler to perform and can be performed on out-patients.

# THE DETECTION OF MICROPROLACTINOMAS

## Sellar radiography

Microprolactinomas do not enlarge the pituitary fossa and in reality plain skull radiographs are only of importance in such cases to exclude a large tumour.

The 'classic' feature on the plain skull radiograph that is said to suggest a microadenoma is the 'double floor' to the pituitary fossa. This is said to be due to a small bulge produced by the tumour growing close to the floor, or even at some distance from it. However,

25

this is a very unreliable sign and appears to be as common in patients who are having their skulls radiographed because of head trauma as in those with a clinical suggestion of a prolactinoma.

The causes of this 'double floor' include:

(1) *Poor radiography;* if the film is not a true lateral one, with the anterior clinoid processes superimposed, even a perfectly flat floor will look double because of the angle of the X-ray beam relative to it.

(2) *A normal central or off-central depression in the sellar floor,* usually associated with the insertion of one or more sphenoidal sinus septa into the floor of the sella.

(3) *A normal slope to the sellar floor* (see below).

(4) *A carotid sulcus.* This is the impression on the side of the upper part of the body of the sphenoid that is fairly common and is caused by the carotid artery; it may even show an anterior curve, easily confused with the sellar floor, corresponding to the anterior curve of the artery to pass medially to the anterior clinoid process.

(5) *Accessory spenoidal sinuses* below and anterior to the sellar floor.

## Sellar tomography

The principle behind the use of sellar tomography in the detection of microprolactinomas is that this technique can show minor changes in the bone of the sellar floor that are supposed to indicate the presence of a small tumour nearby. These changes include focal bulges and erosions, which have to be distinguished from normal variations in this region.

These tomograms are usually obtained by using fairly sophisticated equipment that produces a complex movement of X-ray tube and film to blur out adjacent structures and produce a thin section of bone in focus. The movement is usually hypocycloidal but can be circular or spiral and quite a long X-ray exposure is necessary. The tomographic slice thickness is usually 1 or 2 mm and to cover the whole sella up to 10 or 12 slices may be required in both the axial and the coronal planes. As a result of all this, the radiation dose received by the patient, especially to the radiation-sensitive lenses of the eyes during coronal plane tomography, can be appreciable.

26

Several authors have claimed, over the years, a very close correlation between the positive findings at sellar tomography and their results of transsphenoidal surgery for microprolactinomas[5-7]. However, recently more papers have appeared casting a great deal of doubt on the true value of sellar tomography in the management of patients with suspected microprolactinomas.

The *facts suggesting that sellar tomography is of limited value in detecting microprolactinomas* are:

(1) Quite *marked variations in the configuration of the sellar floor are common*[8,9], on plain radiography or tomography; thus there can be a prominent slope to the floor, a fairly marked central depression and even bone thinning is common normally[10]; these changes can be very difficult to distinguish from pathological features.

(2) *Interpretation of these abnormal findings can be extremely difficult,* even by the most experienced radiologist; in one study[11] two neuroradiologists, with much experience in this field, evaluated the tomograms of a group of patients with suspected microprolactinomas independently and on two separate occasions; they found an inter-observer agreement of only 63–75%, and even the intra-observer agreement was quite poor at 76–85%.

(3) *Post-mortem examination of the pituitary gland, by tomography and microscopy,* has revealed a very poor correlation between the two[12,13]; in one study[12] 32 out of 120 pituitaries were found to contain microadenomas. 41% were prolactinomas but tomography suggested this in only six; a false-negative result in 83%. There was also a false-positive figure of 24%.

(4) *Many normal persons harbour microadenomas in their pituitary glands,* as first described by Costello[14] and confirmed in many other studies since, and as mentioned above in which the prevalence was 27%. These persons, if they were to be tomographed, would be expected to show similar sellar-floor abnormalities making the distinction from those with clinically significant tumours even more difficult.

As a result of all this work, there must be a great deal of doubt about the validity of sellar tomography in the detection of microprolactinomas. We have tried tomography in a large number of cases and found it very disappointing indeed. We found very few definite abnormalities and sometimes when one was identified the surgical exploration revealed no tumour. As a result, we abandoned sellar tomography several years ago and now feel fully vindicated.

## CT scanning

High-definition CT scanning of the sella is becoming the investigation of choice in the detection of microprolactinomas. The technique requires a very sophisticated scanner of the third or fourth generation so that really fine detail of the sella turcica, its contents and the adjacent structures can be seen. The big difference between this type of CT scanning and sellar tomography is that the gland itself is seen, as well as small tumours within it, in addition to indirect features suggesting a mass lesion. Sellar tomography only shows one indirect sign suggesting an intrasellar lesion, namely the rather dubious bony changes in the sellar floor disscused above, that may be at some distance from the tumour itself.

It is generally agreed that the most valuable plane in which to perform these high-definition scans of the sella is the coronal[15]. The sagittal plane is also of value but axial plane scans on their own are of little value as adjacent bone and CSF produce spurious areas of high and low density in the pituitary gland. Coronal-plane scans show the bony sellar floor, as well as the top of the gland, outlined by CSF.

It is possible to carry out the scans in the axial plane and then produce, from these slices, reformatted images in the coronal or sagittal plane, However, the reformatting process tends to degrade the images and the numerous axial plane slices that may be necessary may pass through the eyes. This gives a large radiation dose to the sensitive lenses. We, however, prefer to scan in the direct coronal plane whenever possible, though it is a little more awkward for the patient as the head has to be tilted back into the head-rest to obtain a suitable position. Also, the scanner gantry has to be angled to avoid teeth fillings which produce marked streak artefacts if included in the scan slice, making the scans of little diagnostic value. Sagittal plane scans can be reformatted from these coronal plane scans, if necessary.

Using our pituitary scan protocol we have recently calculated the absorbed radiation dose to the eyes, skin and gonads during pituitary scanning. These measurements were carried out during both axial

28

plane scanning, with the slices passing through the eyes, and direct coronal plane scanning in which the slices are well away from the eyes. The radiation dose to the eyes during axial plane scanning was 45 mGy (4.5 rads or 4500 mrads) but during coronal plane scanning it was only 0.32 mGy (32 mrads), i.e. the dose was 140 times greater for the axial plane scans than for the coronal ones. The dose to the gonads was less than $10\,\mu$Gy; almost unmeasurable.

The scans are obtained with intravenous contrast medium which is infused before and during the scanning procedure. This contrast medium shows the carotid arteries, the arteries in the circle of Willis and the cavernous sinuses due to the circulating opacified blood. It is also taken up by the pituitary gland and the infundibular stalk to a similar degree as the cavernous sinuses. Thus the lateral extent of the gland is difficult to determine, though its top and bottom are well shown. The optic nerves and chiasm do not take up the contrast

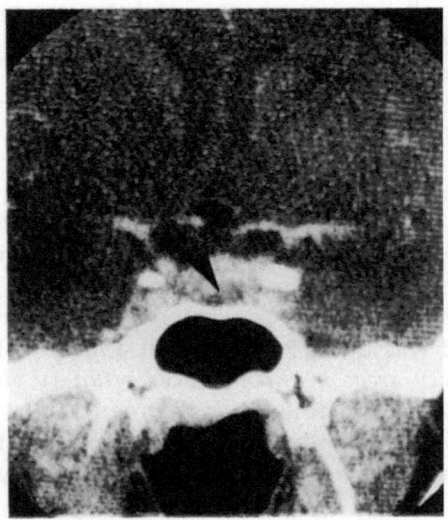

**Figure 1** Direct coronal plane high-definition CT scan of the pituitary gland, showing a microadenoma near the sellar floor (arrowhead); this is seen as a low-density area in the enhanced gland

medium and are quite difficult to see in the suprasellar region. However, the cranial nerves III to VI can usually be seen as negative filling defects in the walls of the cavernous sinuses (Figure 1).

The CT features suggesting a microprolactinoma[15,16] are:

(1) *Enlargement of the pituitary gland,* the normal height being up to 7 mm in the female and a little less in the male.
(2) *Upward convexity* to the upper surface of the gland.
(3) An *area of low density,* the microprolactinoma itself, in the enhanced gland; some microprolactinomas may be the same density as the gland, or even denser, but most appear to be of lower density[17]. Sometimes there is more than one tumour.
(4) *Displacement of the infundibular stalk* away from the low-density prolactinoma; normally the stalk is fairly central.
(5) *Sloping sellar floor* under the tumour.
(6) *Erosion of the floor* in the same region; however, these last two features have to be treated with the same caution as the sellar tomography changes described previously.

Probably, when all or most of these features are present, with the appropriate biochemistry, a microprolactinoma can be fairly confidently diagnosed.

There is some recent evidence suggesting caution in the interpretation of microadenomas in the pituitary gland:

(1) *Normal women may show similar changes.* In a recent study[18] 50 normal women volunteers were scanned in the direct coronal manner and 44% showed an upward convexity to the gland; in addition, 36% showed low densities in the gland that could have been interpreted as a microadenoma and the height of the gland was up to 9.7 mm, with a mean value of 7.1 mm.
(2) *Low-density areas in the enhanced pituitary gland* can be produced by lesions other than microadenomas[19], such as pars intermedia cysts (present in 20% of one postmortem series), infarcts, metastases and even a partial empty sella.

In addition the images produced by the scanner may be 'noisy', with alterations in the gland density which, if they are large, may be easily confused with a small adenoma. Hence some caution has to be used in interpreting these high-definition CT scans, especially until more work has been done on the subject. However, at the moment this type of radiological investigation is the best available for detecting microprolactinomas.

# References

1. Di Chiro, G. and Nelson, K. B. (1962). The volume of the sella turcica. *Am. J. Radiol.*, **87**, 989
2. Hall, K. and McAllister, V. L. (1980). Metrizamide cisternography in pituitary and juxtapituitary lesions. *Radiology*, **134**, 101
3. Hall, K., McGregor, A. M., Scanlon, M. F. and Hall, R. (1980). Metrizamide cisternography in the assessment of pituitary tumour size, with special reference to the demonstration of tumour (prolactinoma) shrinkage on bromocriptine therapy. In Hubinont, P. O. (ed.). *Progress in Reproductive Biology*. Vol. **6**, pp. 232–43. (Basel: Karger)
4. Teasdale, G. and Macpherson, P. (1982). Use of cavernous sinography to detect aneurysms or anomalies of the infraclinoid carotid artery. *J. Neurosurg.*, **57**, 637
5. Richmond, I. L., Newton, T. H. and Wilson, C. B. (1980). Prolactin-secreting pituitary adenomas: correlation of radiographic and surgical findings. *Am. J. Neuroradiol.*, **1**, 13
6. Raji, M. R., Kishore, P. R. S. and Becker, D. P. (1981). Pituitary microadenomas: a radiological–surgical correlative study. *Radiology*, **139**, 95
7. Vezina, J. L. and Sutton, T. J. (1974). Prolactin-secreting pituitary microadenomas. Roentgenologic diagnosis. *Am. J. Radiol.*, **120**, 46
8. Bruneton, J. N., Drouillard, J. P., Sabatier, J. C., Elie, G. P. and Tavernier, J. F. (1979). Normal variants of the sella turcica. Comparison of plain radiographs and tomograms in 200 cases. *Radiology*, **131**, 99
9. Dubois, P. J., Orr, D. P., Hoy, R. J., Herbert, D. L. and Heinz, E. R. (1979). Normal sellar variations in frontal tomograms. *Radiology*, **131**, 105
10. Rhoton, A. L., Harris, F. S. and Renn, W. H. (1977). Microsurgical anatomy of the sellar region and cavernous sinus. *Clin. Neurosurg.*, **24**, 54
11. McLachlan, M. S. and Banna, M. (1979). Observer variations in interpreting radiographs of the pituitary fossa. *Invest. Radiol.*, **14**, 23
12. Burrow, G. N., Wortzman, G., Rewcastle, N. B., Holgate, R. C. and Kovacs, K. (1981). Microadenomas of the pituitary and abnormal sellar tomograms in an unselected autopsy series. *N. Engl. J. Med.*, **304**, 156
13. Turski, P. A., Newton, T. H. and Horten, B. H. (1981). Sellar contour: anatomic–polytomographic correlation. *Am. J. Radiol.*, **137**, 213
14. Costello, R. T. (1936). Subclinical adenoma of the pituitary gland. *Am. J. Pathol.*, **12**, 205
15. Taylor, S. (1982). High resolution computed tomography of the sella. *Radiol. Clin. N. Am.*, **20**, 207
16. Syvertsen, A., Haughton, V. M., Williams, A. L. and Cusick, J. F. (1979). The computed tomographic appearance of the normal pituitary gland and pituitary microadenomas. *Radiology*, **133**, 385
17. Hemminghytt, S., Kalkhoff, R. K., Daniels, D. L., Williams, A. L., Grogan, J. P. and Haughton, V. M. (1983). Computed tomographic study of hormone-secreting microadenomas. *Radiology*, **146**, 65
18. Swartz, J. D., Russell, K. B., Basile, B. A., O'Donnell, P. C. and Popky, G. L. (1983). High resolution computed tomographic appearance of the intrasellar contents in women of childbearing age. *Radiology*, **147**, 115
19. Chambers, E. F., Yurski, P. A., LaMasters, D. and Newton, T. H. (1982). Regions of low density in the contrast-enhanced pituitary gland: normal and pathologic processes. *Radiology*, **144**, 109

# 4

# The outcome of pituitary exploration in patients with hyperprolactinaemic infertility

G. TEASDALE, A. RICHARDS, R. BULLOCK and
J. THOMSON

## INTRODUCTION

The achievement of fertility is a major aim in the treatment of patients with hyperprolactinaemia. When this is considered to be due to a prolactin-producing pituitary adenoma, beneficial effects of treatment may also include removal of the risk that the tumour will enlarge and cause compression on adjacent important structures, either during any subsequent pregnancy or in later life. Of the various methods of treatment that are available, only operation offers the prospect of combining a rapid resolution of hyperprolactinaemia in the short term with the likelihood of long-term avoidance of tumour expansion.

In the last decade, operations on the pituitary gland have become much safer and much more effective. This reflects the swing from performing operations intracranially, gaining access by a standard frontal craniotomy, to approaching the pituitary transsphenoidally and employing the operating microscope. The transsphenoidal route avoids the risks of epilepsy, intracranial haematoma and other neurological complications of intracranial operations and also provides a more direct approach to the face of the gland within the fossa. The operating microscope provides a high illumination and magnification and this has made it possible to identify that in many patients with hypersecretion of pituitary hormones the cause is a small ($< 1$ cm) adenoma contained within an otherwise normal gland. Microsurgical techniques allow the selective removal of the offending lesion, while at the same time preserving normal pituitary tissue. Experience in acromegaly and Cushing's disease has made it clear that the best results are obtained when the tumour is still small – before gross radiological abnormalities appear. The latter herald the enlargement of the tumour to a size such that little normal gland remains – so that a selective operation is more difficult – and also expansion of the tumour into structures outside the pituitary capsule so that the prospects of cure are considerably reduced.

A major problem is the difficulty in the diagnosis of a prolactin-secreting pituitary adenoma while it is small. The problem with the radiological methods is that the first signs are merely minor abnormalities of the fossa on conventional tomograms, or within the tissues of the pituitary gland when studied by modern high-definition CT scanning. Unfortunately, each of these can be seen in between a quarter and a third of otherwise apparently normal young women. Endocrinologically, however, although a very high serum prolactin concentration ($> 4000$ mU l$^{-1}$) is virtually diagnostic of a tumour, when most patients with a microadenoma first present the level is only moderately raised. By itself this does not discriminate a tumour from various 'functional' types of hyperprolactinaemia.

This chapter reports the results in a series of patients who were considered, on the basis of dynamic endocrine tests, to be likely to have a prolactin-secreting pituitary adenoma and who elected to undergo pituitary operation. Most reports of the surgery of prolactinomas have concentrated on the effect on prolactin secretion, often measured only in the immediate post-operative period. The present series is distinctive because patients who desired to conceive have been followed up for long periods and the outcome assessed in respect of pregnancy rate or by their ovulatory status. We also report the course of the 42 pregnancies achieved after operation.

## PATIENTS AND METHODS

The diagnosis of a prolactinoma was based on endocrine criteria: a serum prolactin concentration consistently greater than 360 mU l$^{-1}$ and impaired responses to TRH and metoclopramide, agents that normally produce several-fold increments in serum prolactin concentration[1]. Negative radiological studies[2] did not preclude operation, which was performed by a standard sublabial paraseptal transsphenoidal microsurgical technique. The aim was to identify any tumour, and to remove it; because it is known that adenoma may infiltrate the normal gland, a 1 mm rim of the latter was usually also removed. No patient received radiation therapy before or after operation.

Pituitary function was determined before and after operation according to standard methods and serum prolactin concentrations were determined during and after any pregnancy. Patients with hyperprolactinaemia persisting after operation received bromocriptine treatment, but this was discontinued after conception. In patients who did not conceive, a rise in late cycle of the serum progesterone concentration of more than $20\,\mathrm{mU\,l^{-1}}$ was taken as an index of ovulation.

## RESULTS

The patients' serum prolactin concentrations before operation ranged from 560 to $70\,000\,\mathrm{mU\,l^{-1}}$ with a median value of $2280\,\mathrm{mU\,l^{-1}}$. Only 16 patients had a distinct radiological abnormality; in 11 this was a minor definite change in conventional tomography but in five patients CT scanning showed a tumour with a suprasellar extension. At

**Table 1** Operative findings and postoperative outcome in 40 patients with hyperprolactinaemia and abnormal responses to TRH and metoclopramide

| Adenoma at operation | No. of patients | 'Normal' post-operative PRL* | Fertility | | | |
| --- | --- | --- | --- | --- | --- | --- |
| | | | Operation only | | Operation + BCr | |
| | | | Pregnancy | Ovulation | Pregnancy | Ovulation |
| Micro[†] | 30 | 23 | 18 | 6 | 4 | 2 |
| Macro | 7 | 2 | 1 | – | 4 | – |
| None[‡] | 3 | 1 | 2 | – | 1 | – |

*Normal serum prolactin $< 360\,\mathrm{mU\,l^{-1}}$. Data about ovulatory state were missing in two patients.
†Microadenoma $< 1\,\mathrm{cm}$.
‡Includes one patient with a pituitary granuloma.
BCr = Bromocriptine.

exploration of the pituitary a tumour was found in 37 patients. In seven cases this was a macroadenoma ($> 10\,\mathrm{mm}$). Only one patient developed a potentially serious operative complication; 1 week after operation she developed headache and pyrexia, a lumbar puncture showed a leukocytosis and the presence of *Staphylococcus albus*. This patient recovered fully after antibiotic treatment and has since conceived.

Twenty-six of the 40 women (65%) had a normal basal serum prolactin concentration after operation. The most successfully treated group were patients in whom the tumour was found to be microadenoma, of whom 77% had a normal prolactin level and either conceived or were ovulating after operation (Table 1). After additional bromocriptine treatment all of the remaining patients with a microadenoma became fertile – an overall rate of 100% fertility in this group.

A slightly raised serum prolactin concentration after operation did not preclude fertility. One woman, however, received gonadotrophins before conceiving. Otherwise endocrine deficiency after operation was restricted to two patients both with a large tumour, and persisting diabetes insipidus, and one patient, with impaired reserve before operation, who required cortisone.

Forty-two pregnancies have so far been achieved by 29 women. Of these, only four have miscarried and there were no major congenital malformations:

(1)  Result of pregnancy:
     term delivery, 34; continuing pregnancy, 3; miscarriage, 4; termination, 1.
(2)  Complications:
     multiple pregnancies, 3; antepartum haemorrhage, 1; premature labour, 1; congenital malformation, 0; tumour expansion, 0.

The serum prolactin concentration was normal throughout pregnancy on all but three occasions. This was despite no patient having received bromocriptine treatment during pregnancy. No patient had symptoms during pregnancy that could have been related to an increase in the size of the tumour. On the other hand, two patients whose serum prolactin concentration was normal after operation had recurrent hyperprolactinaemia after delivery, but both have conceived again without further treatment. Another patient, whose serum prolactin concentration had been $1793 \, \mathrm{mU\,l^{-1}}$ after operation, had a level of only $280 \, \mathrm{mU\,l^{-1}}$ after delivery.

In none of the patients who failed to conceive was the reason related to a complication of the operation. Six patients had a normal serum prolactin concentration and four of these who had been tested showed biochemical evidence of ovulation. Two patients, each with a large tumour, had persisting hyperprolactinaemia, despite bromocriptine treatment.

## DISCUSSION

This review shows that an offer of surgery to a patient with biochemical evidence of a prolactinoma results in the majority becoming fertile and also that any subsequent pregnancy is free of complications. The morbidity of the operation is low and no patient has remained infertile as a direct result of a complication of operation.

The relatively favourable results reflect the large proportion of patients who were found to have small tumours, in whom removal of the adenoma was easy to achieve while preserving normal function. Almost all the patients with persisting hyperprolactinaemia had either very large tumours, or a small tumour that had been situated very laterally and had already eroded through the wall of the pituitary and into the cavernous sinus at the time of operation. The large number of small tumours reflects our policy of operating on patients on purely endocrine criteria, but this had the consequence that in three of the 40 patients a tumour was not found. One of the three did have a pituitary granuloma and her prolactin was reduced to normal.

Reports of surgically treated patients include pregnancy rates of 68% in 19 women[3]; 25% in 12 women[4], and 36% in 64 women[5]. Other reports with shorter follow-up bear out the safety and efficacy of the operation in reducing serum prolactin to normal while preserving function in patients with a small adenoma[5,6]. It is clear, therefore, that operation is a more rapid and reliable method than X-ray treatment in the treatment of hyperprolactinaemia due to a prolactin-producing pituitary adenoma. Because operation was followed by freedom of complications in pregnancy, it removes the need for irradiation to guard against this complication occurring in a pregnancy subsequent to bromocriptine therapy, an approach recommended by some authorities.

Reports of medically treated series are difficult to compare with the present series. One reason is that the precise diagnosis in many patients treated medically is uncertain. This is a reflection of the limitations of endocrinological and radiological tests for distinguishing between a tumour and 'functional' hyperprolactinaemia. Moreover, few reports of drug treatment include in their outcome an analysis of the patients who discontinued treatment because of intolerance and who should also be counted as failures of the method.

An operation to explore a normal sized pituitary fossa for a prolactinoma should not be undertaken lightly and is a technically demanding procedure. Nevertheless, these and other reported results suggest that when performed by an experienced surgeon it offers a reasonable alternative to medical treatment. There is clearly a need for further long-term studies of the results of the two approaches.

## Acknowledgements

We thank our many colleagues in the departments of Endocrinology, Obstetrics and Gynaecology, Radiology, and Biochemistry, who have been responsible for the diagnosis and management of the patients included in this report.

## References

1. Cowden, E. A., Thomson, J. A., Doyle, D., Ratcliffe, J. G., Macpherson, P. and Teasdale, G. M. (1979). Tests of prolactin secretion in diagnosis of prolactinomas. *Lancet*, **1**, 1155
2. Teasdale, E., Macpherson, P. and Teasdale, G. (1981). The reliability of radiology in detecting prolactin-secreting pituitary microadenomas. *Br. J. Radiol.*, **54**, 566
3. Landolt, A. M. (1981). Treatment of pituitary prolactinomas: post-operative prolactin and fertility in seventy patients. *Fertil. Steril.*, **35**, 620
4. Guibout, M., Jaquet, P., Lissitzky, J. C., Grisoli, F. and Vincentelli, F. (1978). Resultats de l'exérése transsphenoidale des adenomas hypophysaires secretonits. *Ann. Endocrinol. (Paris)*, **39**, 95
5. Randall, R. V., Laws, E. R., Abboud, C. F., Ebersold, M. J., Kao, P. C. and Scheithauer, B. W. (1983). Transsphenoidal microsurgical treatment of prolactin producing pituitary adenomas. *Mayo Clin. Proc.*, **50**, 108
6. Hardy, J. (1981). Le Prolactinome. *Neurochirugie*, **47**, (Suppl.), 1

# 5
# Medical treatment of prolactinomas

S. FRANKS and H. S. JACOBS

The place of dopamine-receptor agonist drugs in the management of hyperprolactinaemic states has now been firmly established and in the last few years these drugs have been used increasingly as primary treatment in patients with small and large prolactinomas. The purpose of this chapter is not to argue the relative merits of medical and surgical treatment of prolactinomas, but to review the effects of dopaminergic drug therapy in patients with prolactinomas with respect to (1) their effectiveness in restoring normal fertility in hyperprolactinaemic women; (2) their effect on tumour volume; and (3) their effect on the natural history of hyperprolactinaemia. We shall refer, briefly, to the use of low-dose, pulsatile therapy with the luteinizing hormone-releasing hormone (LH-RH) as an alternative means of induction of ovulation in hyperprolactinaemic patients in whom dopaminergic drug treatment has been unsuccessful.

## EFFECTIVENESS OF BROMOCRIPTINE IN HYPERPROLACTINAEMIC AMENORRHOEA

Treatment with bromocriptine rapidly reduces serum prolactin concentrations to normal or near normal and results in ovulatory menses in most women with hyperprolactinaemic anovulation. In our original series of 40 patients (11 with pituitary tumours) on long-term treatment, 36 menstruated and all of these ovulated[1]. Four out of eight patients who had previously received pituitary ablative therapy did not respond – all were gonadotrophin deficient. Seventeen out

39

of 21 infertile patients who received primary treatment with bromocriptine became pregnant; in three of the remaining four there were defined, non-endocrine factors preventing conception. An updated analysis showed that the cumulative conception rate in treated patients was no different from that in the normal population[2]. Recently Bergh and Nillius[3] have reviewed the results of bromocriptine therapy in 120 women with hyperprolactinaemic amenorrhoea (75% of whom had radiological evidence of a prolactinoma). Ovulatory menses occurred in 94% of pre-menopausal women and the pregnancy rate in 54 infertile women was 91%. Thus, in a total of 160 patients (101 with pituitary tumours) from these two series, the overall ovulation rate was 93% and the pregnancy rate 88%.

Treatment with other long-acting dopamine agonists including lisuride, metergoline and pergolide may in the future produce similar results in terms of ovulation rate. Lisuride and metergoline are effective short-acting drugs[4]; pergolide mesylate is a potent, synthetic ergoline derivative with a prolonged action and can therefore be given in a low, once-daily dose[5]. Ovulation occurred in 11 of 14 patients during long-term treatment with pergolide. Side-effects were similar to those of bromocriptine; some patients who had previously had to stop bromocriptine because of side-effects were able to tolerate pergolide but the reverse was also true. Further clinical trials are in progress.

## EFFECTS OF DOPAMINE AGONISTS ON PITUITARY TUMOUR SIZE

One of the most important advances in the management of patients with prolactin-secreting pituitary adenomas is the finding that bromocriptine and other dopamine agonists not only lower prolactin levels but may also cause regression of the tumour (see references 3 and 6 for extensive reviews). This has prompted an increasing number of clinicians to consider bromocriptine as primary therapy in patients with pituitary macroadenomas. A number of case reports, dating from that by Corenblaum et al.[7], showed that bromocriptine treatment was associated with an improvement in the visual-field defects. These reports were followed by studies using radiological criteria to monitor tumour size during treatment and confirmed that there was indeed shrinkage of the prolactinoma. Bergh and Nillius[3] have recently collected data from ten series in which a total of 49 cases have been treated with bromocriptine or lisuride. In 44 (90%) there was evidence of tumour regression during treatment and in many cases the response was very rapid. The reduction in tumour volume seems to be due to a decrease in cell size (the major change being in the cytoplasm) rather than in cell number[8]. Dr A. G. Frantz presented data at the American Endocrine Society in San Francisco (1982) showing that of 105 patients treated in eight series the overall rate of tumour shrinkage was 73%. In the non-responders, tumour growth was noted in five patients in whom there was no significant fall in prolactin and in two of these the tumour increased in size despite a fall in prolactin concentrations. Those patients whose tumours did not shrink on treatment with bromocriptine may in fact have had secondary hyperprolactinaemia associated with a large non-functioning tumour rather than a true prolactinoma. There is no general agreement about the dose of bromocriptine that should be used to shrink tumours but in our experience a dose that is sufficient to keep prolactin levels within the normal range (often as little as 5 mg daily) is also effective in reducing tumour volume.

## FOLLOW-UP OF PATIENTS ON LONG-TERM DOPAMINE AGONIST THERAPY

Limited data are now available concerning the effects of bromocriptine and other dopamine agonists on the natural history of hyperprolactinaemia in patients with and without pituitary tumours. Bergh and Nillius[3] stopped treatment with bromocriptine in 49 patients (37 with pituitary tumours) who had received treatment for at least 12 months. Within 2 months of stopping the drug, prolactin concentrations had returned to pre-treatment levels in 42 (86%) patients. This is consistent with the report from Thorner et al.[9] on two patients in whom rapid return of prolactin levels to pre-treatment concentrations was associated with re-expansion of the tumour. However, the tumour may not necessarily re-grow after bromocriptine treatment is stopped. In one patient in our series bromocriptine was stopped after 6 months of treatment during which there had been significant reduction in the tumour volume. Six months later there has been no radiological recurrence on high-resolution CT scanning in this patient despite the fact that the prolactin concentrations have risen to pre-treatment levels. Five out of 7 patients who had lower post-treatment values were studied by Bergh and Nillius for 1–2 years after therapy was stopped, and in all five prolactin concentrations steadily rose towards pre-treatment levels. Bergh and Nillius noted that most of the patients with prolonged suppression of prolactin following treatment were those with large tumours. Ferrari[4] in a study of 69 patients (most with either microadenomas or idiopathic hyperprolactinaemia) found that although prolactin levels were significantly lower than pre-treatment values after bromocriptine treatment had been stopped, only five resumed ovulatory menses – i.e. a similar remission rate to that observed in an untreated series of hyperprolactinaemic women[10]. This is in contrast to the results following pregnancy in bromocriptine-treated women (*see* below).

## LONG-TERM FOLLOW-UP OF BROMOCRIPTINE-INDUCED PREGNANCIES

A number of groups have shown that prolactin concentrations following bromocriptine-induced pregnancies may be lower than the pre-treatment levels[3,11-13]. Bergh and Nillius reported persistent reduction in prolactin concentrations in 19 out of 28 women (a mixture of tumour and non-tumour patients), and three of these patients resumed spontaneous ovulatory menstruation.

We have recently reviewed our own series of 27 patients with normal pituitary X-rays who had previously been treated with bromocriptine and in whom treatment was discontinued. Sixty per cent of women with amenorrhoea and normal pituitary X-rays whose prolactin concentrations were less than $2000\,mU\,l^{-1}$ were cured, in the sense that basal prolactin levels were normal and ovulatory cycles resumed after stopping bromocriptine[12]. When these patients were tested with TRH before treatment with bromocriptine the response of prolactin was impaired, i.e. showing a similar abnormality in regulation of prolactin secretion as in other hyperprolactinaemic patients (Figure 1). Thus although most patients with hyperprolactinaemia will require further treatment with bromocriptine, a significant proportion of those with normal pituitary X-rays appear to be cured following pregnancy. This may represent persistent shrinkage of a small prolactinoma or perhaps resolution of true 'functional' hyperprolactinaemia.

# INDUCTION OF OVULATION WITH LOW-DOSE PULSATILE LH-RH IN HYPERPROLACTINAEMIC WOMEN

A number of studies have shown that the mechanism of the reproductive disorder in hyperprolactinaemia is related to an abnormality in the hypothalamic regulation of gonadotrophin secretion[14-16] which manifests itself as a grossly abnormal pattern of pulsatile LH secretion[17,18]. The importance of the hypothalamic abnormality is illustrated by the fact that ovulation can be induced in women with

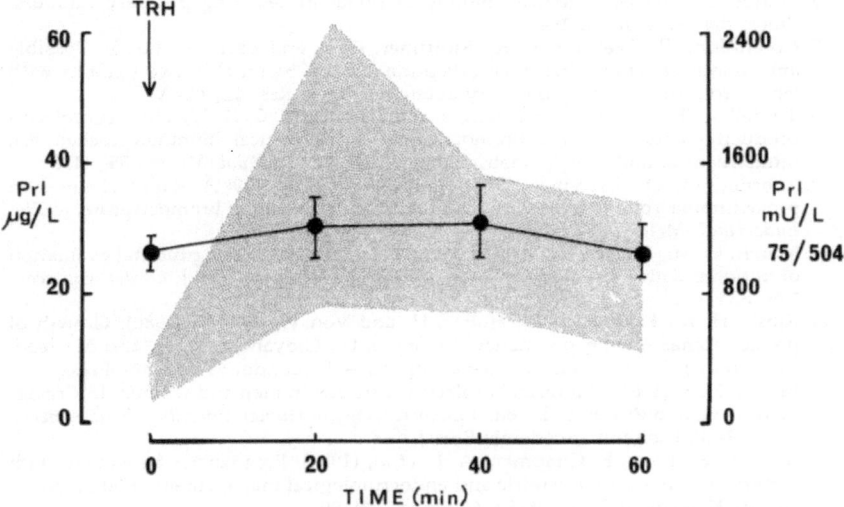

**Figure 1** The prolactin response to 200 μg of TRH prior to therapy in those patients who subsequently underwent cure. The shaded area indicates the range of responses in normal women

persistent hyperprolactinaemia by low-dose pulsatile LH-RH[19]. This is also of practical importance since this form of treatment may be used to induce ovulation in women in whom dopamine agonists have failed either because of unacceptable side-effects or (as in a very few patients) because the hyperprolactinaemia appears 'resistant' to bromocriptine.

## References

1. Franks, S., Jacobs, H. S., Hull, M. G. R., Steele, S. J. and Nabarro, J. D. N. (1977). Management of hyperprolactinaemic amenorrhoea. *Br. J. Obstet. Gynaecol.*, **84**, 241

2. Hull, M. G. R., Savage, P. A. and Jacobs, H. S. (1979). Investigations and treatment of amenorrhoea resulting in normal fertility. *Br. Med. J.*, **1**, 1257
3. Bergh, T. and Nillius, S. J. (1982). Prolactinomas: follow up of medical treatment. In Molinatti, G. M. (ed.) *A Clinical Problem: Microprolactinoma*. pp. 115–30. (Oxford: Excerpta Medica)
4. Ferrari, C., Mattei, A., Rampini, P., *et al.* (1982). Long-term effects of drug treatment on hyperprolactinaemic disorders: a study after discontinuation of bromocriptine and metergoline. In Molinatti, G. M. (ed.) *A Clinical Problem: Microprolactinoma*. pp. 141–48. (Oxford: Excerpta Medica)
5. Franks, S., Horrocks, P. M., Lynch, S. S., Butt, W. R. and London, D. R. (1983). Effectiveness of pergolide mesylate in long term treatment of hyperprolactinaemia. *Br. Med. J.*, **286**, 1177
6. Nillius, S. J. (1980). Medical therapy of prolactin secreting pituitary tumours. *Progr. Reprod. Biol.*, **6**, 194
7. Corenblum, B., Webster, B. R., Mortimer, C. B. and Ezrin, C. (1975). Possible antitumour effect of 2-bromoergocryptine (CB-154 Sandoz) in two patients with large prolactin-secreting pituitary adenomas. *Clin. Res.*, **23**, 614A
8. Tindall, G. T., Kovacs, K., Horvath, E. and Thorner, M. O. (1982). Human prolactin producing adenomas and bromocriptine: a histological immunocytochemical, ultrastructural and morphometric study. *J. Clin. Endocrinol. Metab.*, **55**, 1178
9. Thorner, M. O., Perryman, R., Rogol, A. D., *et al.* (1981). Rapid changes in prolactinoma volume after withdrawal and reinstitution of bromocriptine. *J. Clin. Endocrinol. Metab.*, **53**, 480
10. March, C. M., Kletzky, O. A., Davajan, V., *et al.*, (1981). Longitudinal evaluation of patients with untreated prolactin-secreting adenomas. *Am. J. Obstet. Gynecol.*, **139**, 835
11. Rjosk, H. K., Fahlbusch, R., Huber, H. and Von Werder, K. (1980). Growth of prolactinomas during pregnancy. In Faglia, G., Giovanelli, M. A. and Macleod, R. M. (eds.) *Pituitary Microadenomas*. pp. 535–41. (London: Academic Press)
12. Jacobs, H. S. (1981). Abnormal prolactin secretion in men and women. In Crosignani, P. G. and Rubin, B. L. (eds.) *Endocrinology of Human Infertility: New Aspects*. pp. 129–38. (London: Academic Press)
13. Randall, S., Lang, I., Chapman, A. J., *et al.* (1982). Pregnancies in women with hyperprolactinaemia: obstetric and endocrinological management of 50 pregnancies in 37 women. *Br. J. Obstet. Gynaecol.*, **89**, 20
14. Glass, M. R., Shaw, R. W., Butt, W. R., Logan Edwards, R. and London, D. R. (1975). An abnormality of oestrogen feedback in amenorrhoea–galactorrhoea. *Br. Med. J.*, **3**, 274
15. Jacobs, H. S., Franks, S., Murray, M. A. F., Hull, M. G. R., Steele, S. J. and Nabarro, J. D. N. (1976). Clinical and endocrine features of hyperprolactinaemic amenorrhoea. *Clin. Endocrinol.*, **5**, 439
16. Aono, T., Miyake, A., Schioji, T., Kinugasa, T., Onishi, T. and Kurachi, K. (1976). Impaired LH release following exogenous estrogen administration in patients with amenorrhoea galactorrhoea syndrome. *J. Clin. Endocrinol. Metab.*, **42**, 696
17. Bohnet, H. G., Dahlen, H. G., Wuttke, W. and Schneider, H. P. G. (1976). Hyperprolactineamic anovulatory syndrome. *J. Clin. Endocrinol. Metab.*, **●**, 132
18. Moult, P. J. A., Rees, L. H. and Besser, G. M. (1982). Pulsatile gonadatrophin secretion in hyperprolactinaemic amenorrhea and the response to bromocriptine therapy. *Clin. Endocrinol.*, **16**, 153
19. Leyendecker, G., Struve, T. and Plotz, E. J. (1980). Induction of ovulation with chronic intermittent (pulsatile) administration of LHRH in women with hypothalamic and hyperprolactinaemic amenorrhoea. *Arch. Gynaecol.*, **229**, 172

# 6
# Surveillance of Parlodel (bromocriptine) in pregnancy and offspring

P. KRUPP and I. TURKALJ

---

Hyperprolactinaemic conditions often lead to infertility, particularly in female patients. Before the therapeutic potential of Parlodel (bromocriptine) was investigated in women suffering from such endocrinological disorders, the drug was carefully studied in animals. The results of the comprehensive toxicological studies, which were performed in various animal species including the stump-tailed monkey, indicate that Parlodel is neither mutagenic, embryotoxic or teratogenic[1]. This information is important in so far as women with infertility secondary to hyperprolactinaemia may become pregnant when treated with Parlodel[2,3] and medication is likely to continue after conception, if only until the patient becomes aware that she is pregnant or the diagnosis is confirmed. It was, therefore, essential to ascertain in humans whether this drug does not affect the course and the outcome of pregnancy or the postnatal development of the offspring when continued after conception. To investigate this problem, a stepwise procedure consisting of three surveys was set up. The first two surveys were aimed at gathering information on the progress and outcome of pregnancies in women treated with Parlodel during gestation. The data collection of the first study was based on spontaneous reporting. The results of this survey have already been published[4]. The second survey consisted of an intensive monitoring project; with this

45

approach it was possible to obtain information from the participating clinics about all pregnant women being treated with Parlodel. The third step was a follow-up survey of the postnatal development of infants exposed to Parlodel *in utero*. This investigation was performed because bromocriptine, the active ingredient of Parlodel, crosses the placental barrier.

## SPONTANEOUS REPORTING

Clinicians known to treat women suffering from hyperprolactinaemic conditions with Parlodel were invited to cooperate in a pregnancy survey. Special report forms were provided for obtaining the relevant information about the indication and dosage of bromocriptine, on the course, duration and outcome of pregnancy as well as on the status of the newborn babies, including sex, weight and length. At first, most reports came from clinicians who had been involved in the clinical evaluation of Parlodel before the product was marketed; the standard of record keeping was high, as virtually every patient could be followed up on an individual basis. Later, when the survey was extended and physicians of more than 30 countries participated, individual monitoring was no longer possible. Consequently, in some cases the reports were incomplete. For obvious reasons a control group could not be included.

Information was obtained on 1410 pregnancies in 1335 patients treated with Parlodel after conception, from 1973 to 1980. In 82% of the cases, Parlodel was given for the treatment of amenorrhoea or luteal insufficiency, while in 18% pituitary tumours, including acromegaly, were reported as the primary diagnosis.

The median age of the patients was 29 years, the oldest being 42 years. The daily dose of Parlodel ranged from 1.25 to 40 mg, the median daily dose being 5 mg. The median duration of Parlodel medication after conception amounted to 21 days. However, in a few patients the drug was already discontinued 1 day after conception. Nine patients were treated throughout the period of gestation. The course of pregnancy was uneventful in these patients; all were delivered healthy babies with no abnormalities.

Spontaneous abortion occurred in 11.2% of the pregnancies; this figure includes nine missed abortions. This percentage compares favourably with those of 10–15% quoted in the literature for a normal population[5]. There was no evidence that the occurrence of spontane-

46

ous abortion was influenced by the Parlodel dosage, the duration of treatment after conception or withdrawal of the drug. Moreover, no consistency could be found with respect to the interval between discontinuation of Parlodel and the occurrence of abortion such as might be expected if cessation of therapy was associated with hormonal changes, leading to abortion.

Of the 1410 pregnancies 86% resulted in births, 97.8% were single births. Twenty-four patients delivered twins and two patients triplets. Two mothers with twins and one mother with triplets were receiving concomitant treatment with clomiphene or gonadotrophin. If these multiplets are disregarded, the corrected incidence of twin births (1.8%) is somewhat but not significantly increased when compared with a normal population[6]. Likewise, in two other surveys of babies born to Parlodel-treated mothers, multiplets were observed only when clomiphene or gonadotrophins had also been prescribed concurrently[7,8]. The mean birth weights of both, single births and twins, were comparable with those in a normal population.

Minor congenital malformations or abnormalities were noted in 2.5% of the babies. Most often they consisted of congenital dislocation of the hip or talipes. In addition to certain organ deficiencies such as hydrocephalus, pulmonary atresia or renal agenesis, the major malformations, observed in 1% of the babies, included two cases of Down's syndrome. However, in a special study performed in babies born to Parlodel-treated mothers, no drug-induced chromosomal defects could be found[9]. Moreover, exploratory data analysis revealed no difference with respect to the daily dose, the duration of treatment after conception, or the total intake of Parlodel between mothers who gave birth to normal children and those who had children with malformations.

## INTENSIVE MONITORING

The second survey of Parlodel in pregnancy, which was started in 1979, is still ongoing and is scheduled to last until the end of September 1983. This intensive monitoring project is being conducted in 35 clinics in 12 different countries. In these clinics each patient receiving Parlodel after conception was registered and followed up until delivery. Therefore, under-reporting and other drawbacks of the first survey, based on spontaneous reporting, could be prevented. Again, special patient sheets were designed for data collection. The

47

survey included a comparative group consisting of babies with malformations, who were born at the participating clinics to mothers not treated with Parlodel during the monitoring period. However, at some of the clinics in one country the information on the babies, serving as controls, could be obtained only via the national malformation register and not with the special design forms. During the progress of the study it also became evident that at some clinics, the control babies were not examined by the same physician and not as carefully as the babies exposed to Parlodel *in utero*. Therefore, only a limited comparison between the two groups is possible, and in particular, with respect to minor malformations and abnormalities.

The available information on 563 pregnancies in Parlodel-treated mothers confirmed the results obtained in the first survey: the main indication for Parlodel medication was amenorrhoea; only about 19% of the patients received the drug for a pituitary tumour or for acromegaly. The median age of the mothers was 28 years, the daily dose of Parlodel 5 mg and the median duration of medication after conception 24 days. However, the incidence of spontaneous abortion and the corrected incidence of twin births were 8.8% and 1.4% respectively, somewhat lower than in the first survey. No triplets were reported. Likewise, the malformation rate, calculated for the babies born to Parlodel-treated mothers, was also lower in this intensive monitoring study. The incidence for major malformations was 1.7% and that for minor malformations 0.8%. No clustering of a special type of birth defect could be recognized. With the exception of three babies with talipes and two babies with ventricular septal defects – malformations relatively often seen in the normal population – the other types of birth defects noted in the exposed babies were observed just once each, and no organ system was preferentially affected.

## POSTNATAL DEVELOPMENT

In the third survey, which consisted of a follow-up investigation, children exposed to Parlodel *in utero* were examined by paediatricians according to a defined questionnaire. The main difficulty encountered was the enrolment of these children, as many lived far away from the clinics where their mothers had been treated; others had moved with their families and they could no longer be traced.

Up to now information on 212 Caucasian children is available.

Their age at examination ranged from 5 to 63 months. Most had been exposed to Parlodel *in utero* during the first 4 weeks after conception. One child was exposed throughout gestation. In 82% of this cohort weight and height were within the normal range; 12 and 10%, respectively, exceeded the 95th percentile. The clinical findings noted in some of these children were scattered throughout all organ systems; they included abnormalities already present at birth, functional disorders such as constipation, conditions such as atopic dermatitis or viral infections such as varicella. Findings of these types are frequently observed in children of this age. No specific pattern of abnormal postnatal development could be recognized. These results have recently been confirmed with a follow-up study on 134 Japanese infants born to Parlodel-treated mothers[8].

## DISCUSSION AND CONCLUSION

The results obtained in the first two surveys are similar and indicate that there is no special risk for the fetus inherent in Parlodel therapy during pregnancy, as the rates of spontaneous abortion, multiple pregnancy and, in particular, of malformations were not increased in patients treated with this drug during gestation.

According to a recent comprehensive review of the literature, the congenital malformation rates published ranged from 1 to 9%[10]. The rates of 3.5 and 2.5% observed in this surveillance lie well within these limits. Moreover, the classification of malformations encountered, according to the organ systems affected, shows a distribution similar to that described by Heinonen *et al.*[11]. The data gleaned from the intensive monitoring study is probably more realistic, as in this survey every patient treated with Parlodel after conception was recorded. The information based on spontaneous reporting – the method used in the first survey – tended to overestimate negative effects.

The results obtained in the follow-up study indicate that exposure to Parlodel *in utero* does not influence postnatal development.

Summing up, no adverse effect of Parlodel medication during pregnancy could be recognized by this comprehensive surveillance which was conducted over a decade. However, as Parlodel diminishes prolactin secretion in the fetus and as the occurrence of spontaneous abortion is not enhanced by interruption of treatment, it is recommended that Parlodel be stopped as soon as pregnancy is confirmed unless there is a definite indication for it to be continued.

## References

1. Richardson, B. P., Turkalj, I. and Flückiger, E. (1983). Bromocriptine. In Lawrence, D. R. (ed.) *Safety and Testing of New Drugs, Prediction and Performance.* (In press)
2. Thorner, M. O., Besser, G. M. and Jones, A. (1975). Bromocriptine treatment of female infertility: Report of 13 pregnancies. *Br. Med. J.*, **iv,** 964
3. Franks, S., Jacobs, H. S. and Hull, M. G. (1977). Management of hyperprolactin-aemic amenorrhoea. *Br. J. Obstet. Gynaecol.*, **84,** 241
4. Turkalj, I., Braun, P. and Krupp, P. (1982). Surveillance of bromocriptine in pregnancy. *J. Am. Med. Assoc.*, **247,** 1589
5. Helbing, W. (1966). Pathologie der Frühschwangerschaft. In Döderlein, G. and Wulf, K.-H. (eds.) *Klinik der Frauenheilkunde und Geburtshilfe.* Vol. 5, p. 22. (Munich: Urban and Schwarzenberg)
6. Deutsche Forschungsgemeinschaft (German Research Council) (1977). *Schwanger-schaftsverlauf und Kindsentwicklung.* p. 86. (Boppard, W. Germany: Harald Boldt.)
7. Thorner, M. O., Edwards, C. R. W., Charlesworth, M., Dacie, J. E., Moult, P. J. A., Rees, L. H., Jones, A. E. and Besser, G. M. (1979). Pregnancy in patients presenting with hyperprolactinaemia. *Br. Med. J.*, **2,** 771
8. Kurachi, K. (1983). A follow-up of infants born to mothers treated with bromocrip-tine: Results obtained by the Japanese Study Group on Hyperprolactinaemia. (In press)
9. Schellekens, L. A., Snuiverink, H. and van den Berghe, H. (1977). Chromosomal pattern of children born after induction of ovulation with bromocriptine. *Drug Res.*, **27,** 2151
10. Hauser, G. A. (1980). Bromocriptine in pregnancy: No teratogenic risk. *Med. Trib.*, **15,** 45
11. Heinonen, O. P., Slone, D. and Shapiro, S. (1977). *Birth Defects and Drugs in Pregnancy.* (Littleton, Ill.: Publishing Sciences Group)

# 7
# Prolactinomas in pregnancy

T. BERGH AND S. J. NILLIUS

It is well known that women with pituitary tumours may develop symptoms from tumour enlargement during pregnancy[1]. To decrease the risk of pregnancy-induced tumour growth some authorities recommend that women with prolactinomas should have their tumour treated by irradiation or surgery before pregnancy. However, the effect of X-ray therapy on prolactinomas is slow and often ineffective[2]. Furthermore, irradiation does not completely prevent the risk of tumour growth during pregnancy[1]. Pituitary microsurgery has to be performed by very experienced neurosurgeons; and in inexpert hands it can have disastrous results[2]. Because of the poor outcome of pituitary microsurgery in women with prolactinomas, Nabarro[2] in a recent review concluded that bromocriptine should be used as much as possible. The risk for serious irreversible complications due to growth of prolactinomas during pregnancy induced by bromocriptine has been exaggerated[1]. Today primary medical therapy with dopamine agonists is given to most infertile women with prolactin-secreting pituitary adenomas.

## PRIMARY BROMOCRIPTINE TREATMENT OF INFERTILE WOMEN WITH PROLACTINOMAS

The risk that women with prolactinomas develop symptoms from tumour enlargement during pregnancy has previously been estimated to vary between 5 and 25%[1]. In nine recent studies 268 hyperprolactinaemic women with untreated prolactinomas experienced a total

51

of 300 term pregnancies after treatment with dopamine agonists, mostly bromocriptine (Table 1). In only four of these pregnancies were there severe complications that had to be treated. All four patients were successfully treated by bromocriptine or surgery during the pregnancy. No evidence of tumour growth was found during pregnancy or at the postpartum evaluation in 281 of the 300 pregnancies (94%).

**Table 1** Number of pregnancies and tumour complication in nine series of hyperprolactinaemic infertile women given primary dopamine agonist therapy. Patients who have had tumour therapy with surgery or irradiation are not included

| Reference | No. of patients | No. of pregnancies | Prolactinoma complications during pregnancy | | Total no. of patients | Comments |
|---|---|---|---|---|---|---|
| | | | Visual impairment | Radiologic progression | | |
| 3,4 | 30 | 33 | 1 | 4 | 5 | 14 patients with macroadenomas |
| 5 | 38 | 38 | 1 | 4 | 4 | |
| 6 | 25 | 25 | 0 | 0 | 0 | Macroadenomas not treated |
| 7 | 15 | 17 | 0 | 1 | 1 | |
| 8 | 61 | 79 | 1 | 0 | 1 | |
| 9 | 30 | 40 | 0 | 1 | 1 | |
| 10 | 48 | 47 | 0 | 0 | 0 | Macroadenomas not treated |
| 11 | 19 | 19 | 1 | 7 | 7 | |
| Total | 268 | 300 | 4 | 17 | 19 | |

We have given primary bromocriptine therapy to 68 infertile women with hyperprolactinaemia. Forty-eight had an asymmetric pituitary fossa. The sellar asymmetry was pronounced in 24 of the women (asymmetry > 3 mm). None of the patients had received prior tumour therapy with irradiation or surgery. Empty sella or suprasellar extension of the pituitary tumour was excluded by computerized tomography (CAT scan). The mean prolactin level before treatment was $65 \mu g \, l^{-1}$ (range $24–144 \mu g \, l^{-1}$) in the women with a normal sella and $101 \mu g \, l^{-1}$ (range $30–1470 \mu g \, l^{-1}$) in the women with radiological changes of the pituitary fossa. The bromocriptine treatment resulted in 90 pregnancies in the 68 women (69 term pregnancies, 11 induced and 10 spontaneous abortions).

Evidence of tumour growth during pregnancy was found in five women. One woman developed visual field defects in the last trimester of the pregnancy. Reinstitution of bromocriptine restored normal vision and the pregnancy could continue to term. Postpartum sellar X-ray showed destruction of the sella[12]. In four other women the sellar X-ray had changed during the pregnancy. One of the women complained of headache from the second trimester but had normal visual fields. The other three women had clinically uneventful pregnancies. The subtle radiographic changes in these four women were probably caused by tumour growth during pregnancy. However, it is not known whether similar changes may occur during pregnancy in healthy women. In three of the four women, radiological regression occurred within 2 years after the delivery[3]. One of the patients in our series had radiological signs of tumour enlargement despite a normal sellar X-ray before pregnancy. There are other case reports in the literature indicating that patients with normal sellar X-rays might develop severe tumour complications during pregnancy[1]. Such a patient was recently referred to us. Before pregnancy her sellar X-ray was judged to be normal. In the last trimester of pregnancy she developed visual field defects and decreased visual acuity. Vision rapidly returned to normal when bromocriptine was reinstituted during the pregnancy. The tumour regression was verified by CAT scan[13]. Thus, a normal pituitary fossa X-ray does not exclude the risk of pregnancy-induced pituitary tumour growth. A pretreatment CAT scan should be performed in all infertile women with hyperprolactinaemia.

## MANAGEMENT OF WOMEN WITH PROLACTINOMAS DURING PREGNANCY

The infertile woman with hyperprolactinaemia should be fully informed about the possibility of tumour enlargement during pregnancy. If she develops symptoms that may be associated with tumour growth, she should be referred to a specialist familiar with the rare complications. During pregnancy, the patient should be followed up with monthly visual field examinations for earliest possible detection of visual impairment.

If symptoms of rapid tumour enlargement occur during pregnancy they can be treated with favourable outcome for mother and child. The two patients we have seen with visual field defects during pregnancy have both rapidly responded to bromocriptine with normalization of vision. In the literature there are other case reports in which prolactinoma complications during pregnancy have been successfully treated with bromocriptine[14]. Reinstitution of bromocriptine should therefore be the treatment of choice, if symptoms of tumour expansion occur. Should this therapy fail other treatment alternatives are available[1].

It has been suggested that bromocriptine treatment should be maintained throughout pregnancy to prevent tumour enlargement. Bromocriptine has not been shown to have any adverse effects on the pregnancy or the fetus[15]. However, the incidence of serious tumour complications during pregnancy is very low. We therefore do not think that it is justified to give prophylactic medical treatment with bromocriptine to all pregnant women with hyperprolactinaemia.

## POSTPARTUM MANAGEMENT OF PATIENTS WITH PROLACTINOMAS

Some authors have discouraged patients with prolactinomas from breast feeding in order to decrease the stimulatory effect on the pituitary lactotrophs[11]. All our patients with prolactinoma have breast fed without any untoward effects being observed. One of the patients with visual field defects during pregnancy could breast feed normally when bromocriptine therapy was discontinued 2 days postpartum[13]. In this patient further tumour regression could be verified radiologically during the period of lactation. In our opinion there is therefore no reason to withhold hyperprolactinaemic women from the advantages of breast feeding.

After pregnancy and lactation many hyperprolactinaemic patients have decreased serum prolactin levels in comparison with the pretreatment values. In some women spontaneous ovulatory menstruations have even returned[7,14]. In our present series 31 of the women with sellar asymmetries have had their prolactin levels measured after the bromocriptine-induced pregnancies. In these women the mean prolactin level decreased from 110 to $76 \mu g\,l^{-1}$ ($p < 0.05$). Only three of the women had a higher prolactin level after pregnancy than before. Thus it is very uncommon for pregnancy to make the hyperprolactinaemic condition worse.

## CONCLUDING REMARKS

The incidence of complications caused by growth of prolactinomas during pregnancy is low. The risk that pregnancy-induced tumour expansion leads to severe and permanent sequelae is very small in carefully supervised patients. In infertile hyperprolactinaemic patients without evidence of extrasellar growth of a prolactinoma, primary medical therapy with dopamine agonists is the treatment of choice.

## References

1. Nillius, S. J., Bergh, T. and Larsson, S.-G. (1980). Pituitary tumours and pregnancy. In Derome, P. J., Jedynak, C. P. and Peillon, F. (eds.) *Pituitary Adenomas. Biology, Physiopathology and Treatment*, pp. 103–11. (France: Asclepios Publishers)
2. Nabarro, J. D. N. (1982). Pituitary prolactinomas. *Clin. Endocrinol.*, **17**, 129
3. Bergh, T., Nillius, S. J., Larsson, S.-G. and Wide, L. (1981). Effects of bromocriptine-induced pregnancy on prolactin-secreting pituitary tumours. *Acta Endocrinol.*, **98**, 333
4. Bergh, T., Nillius, S. J., Enoksson, P., Larsson, S.-G. and Wide, L. (1982). Bromocriptine-induced pregnancies in women with large prolactinomas. *Clin. Endocrinol.*, **17**, 625
5. Crosignani, P. G., Ferrari, C., Scarduelli, C., Picciotti, M. C., Caldara, R. and Malinverni, A. (1981). Spontaneous and induced pregnancies in hyperprolactinemic women. *Obstet. Gynecol.*, **58**, 708
6. Jewelewicz, R. and Van de Wiele, R. L. (1980). Clinical course and outcome of pregnancy in twenty-five patients with pituitary microadenomas. *Am. J. Obstet. Gynecol.*, **136**, 339
7. Nyboe Andersen, A., Starup, J., Tabor, A., Kålund Jensen, H. and Westergaard, J. G. (1983). The possible prognostic value of serum prolactin increment during pregnancy in hyperprolactinaemic patients. *Acta Endocrinol.*, **102**, 1
8. Pepperell, R. J. (1981). Prolactin and reproduction. *Fertil. Steril.*, **35**, 267
9. Randall, S., Laing, I., Chapman, A. J., Shalet, S. M., Beardwell, C. G., Kelly, W. F. and Davies, D. (1982). Pregnancies in women with hyperprolactinaemia: obstetric and endocrinological management of 50 pregnancies in 37 women. *Br. J. Obstet. Gynaecol.*, **89**, 20
10. Rjosk, H.-K., Fahlbusch, R. and von Werder, K. (1982). Influence of pregnancies on prolactinomas. *Acta Endocrinol.*, **100**, 337
11. Shewchuck, A. B., Adamson, G. D., Lessard, P. and Ezrin, C. (1980). The effect of pregnancy on suspected pituitary adenomas after conservative management of ovulation defects associated with galactorrhea. *Am. J. Obstet. Gynecol.*, **136**, 659
12. Bergh, T., Nillius, S. J. and Wide, L. (1978). Clinical course and outcome of pregnancies in amenorrhoeic women with hyperprolactinaemia and pituitary tumours. *Br. Med. J.*, **i**, 875
13. Bergh, T., Nillius, S. J., Enoksson, P. E. and Wide, L. (1983). Bromocriptine regression of suprasellar extension of a prolactinoma during pregnancy. (Submitted for publication)
14. Bergh, T. and Nillius, S. J. (1982). Prolactinomas – follow-up of medical treatment. In Molinatti, G. M. (ed.) *A Clinical Problem: Microprolactinoma. Diagnosis and Treatment.* pp. 115–30. (Amsterdam: Excerpta Medica)
15. Turkalj, I., Braun, P. and Krupp, P. (1982). Surveillance of bromocriptine in pregnancy. *J. Am. Med. Assoc.*, **247**, 1589

# Index

abortion, spontaneous and bromocriptine 46–8
acromegaly 14, 46
adenoma, diagnosis of pituitary 22
amenorrhoea
  and bromocriptine 39, 40
  hyperprolactinaemic 9

breast feeding and prolactinomas 54
bromocriptine 10, 11
  and hyperprolactinaemic amenorrhoea 39, 40
  indications 46, 48
  -induced pregnancy, follow-up 42
  long-term therapy and prolactin levels 41, 42
  postnatal effects 48, 49
  pregnancy effects 46, 47, 51–5
  pregnancy outcome 47, 48
  pregnancy rate 40
  prolactinoma treatment 35
  prophylactic in pregnancy 54
  side-effects, assessment 45, 54
  tumour enlargement in pregnancy 51
  tumour shrinkage 41
  visual field defects 40, 52, 53

cerebral angiography and macroprolactinoma removal 24
computerized tomography (CT, CAT)
  and basal cisternography 25
  and eye radiation dose 29
  microadenoma 28–30
  microprolactinoma, features 29
  interpretation 29, 30
  pituitary scanning 9, 10, 23, 24, 28–30, 52, 53

sella visualization 28
congenital abnormalities and bromocriptine use 47
contrast media, basal cisternography 25

domperidone tests 14, 16, 17
dopaminergic agonist and precursor tests 14
  prolactinoma shrinkage 40, 41
  serum prolactin in hyperprolactinaemia 17
dopaminergic drug test 14
  prolactin response and hyperprolactinaemia type 18, 19
double floor, causes 25, 26

hyperprolactinaemia *see also* infertility
  basal serum prolactin levels and causes 15–18
  hypothalamic 14, 18
  idiopathic 13, 18
  micro- and macroprolactinoma 13, 14, 18
  oestrogen deficiency 9

infertility, hyperprolactinaemic and pituitary exploration 33–5

lisuride 40
luteinizing hormone-releasing hormone (LH-RH)
  adverse reactions 43
  ovulation induction in hyperprolactinaemia 43

macroprolactinoma 13, 14, 18
  neuroradiological detection 22–5
  and sella size 22
metergoline 40
metoclopramide test 35
microprolactinoma 13, 14, 18
  features in CT scanning and inter-
    pretation 29, 30
  incidence 27
  neuroradiological detection 25–30
  and sella 22
  treatment success and fertility 36

neuroradiology of prolactinomas 21–30
  see also individual techniques and
    tumours
  choice of technique 21
  localization 22

ovulation, LH-RH induced in hyperprolactinaemia 43

Parlodel see bromocriptine
pergolide mesylate 40
  and ovulation 40
postnatal development and bromocriptine use 48, 49
pregnancy
  bromocriptine effects 46–8
  bromocriptine-induced, follow-up 42
  multiple 47, 49
  outcome and microprolactinoma
    treatment 36
  rates and pituitary surgery 37
  tumour enlargement and bromocrip-
    tine 51, 52
  tumour regression following 53
prolactinoma
  complications in pregnancy 52
  diagnosis 9, 34 see also macro- and
    microprolactinoma
  incidence 9
  normal patients 27, 34
  management in pregnancy 53, 54

neuroradiology 21–30
postpartum management 54
treatment and assessment 10
  medical 39–43
  surgical 34–7

radiography
  pituitary fossa 'double floor' 25, 26
  sellar 25, 26

sella
  aneurysms 24
  causes of enlarged 22, 23
  investigations 13
  radiography 22, 23, 25, 26
  tomography 23, 26–8
serum prolactin levels 13, 34
  bromocriptine treatment in preg-
    nancy 52, 54
  and hyperprolactinaemia aetiology
    15, 35
sinus venography, cavernous 25
sulpiride tests 14
  prolactin response in hyperprolactin-
    aemia 16, 17
surgery, pituitary
  outcome and pregnancy 34, 36, 37
  techniques and risks 33, 34, 51

tomography
  assessment in microprolactinoma de-
    tection 27
  and microprolactinoma detection
    26–8
  sellar, technique 26
  and surgery assessment 27
TRH test 14, 35
  serum prolactin in hyperprolactin-
    aemia 16
TSH test and prolactin levels in hyperprolactinaemia 18

visual impairment 40, 52, 53
  bromocriptine response 53